SPINAL STENOSIS DIET COOKBOOK FOR BEGINNERS

Deliciously Simple Anti-Inflammatory Recipes for Symptom Alleviation, Osteoporosis Prevention, and Improved Muscle Strength

Marian Elbert, RDN

COPYRIGHT PAGE

Table of Contents

PART I: Introduction to Spinal Stenosis and Diet

Spinal stenosis happens when the spaces in the spine narrow and create pressure on the spinal cord and nerve roots. The spinal cord is a bundle of nerves that comes out of the base of the brain and runs down the center of the spine. The nerve roots branch out from the cord. The narrowing usually occurs over time and involves one or more areas of the spine:

The spinal canal, the hollow space in the center of each vertebrae (bones in the spine that protect the spinal cord); the spinal cord and nerve roots run through the spinal canal.

The space at the base or roots of nerves branching out from the spinal cord.

The openings between vertebrae, through which nerves leave the spine and go to other parts of the body.

Spinal stenosis can affect anyone, but it's most common in people over the age of 50.

The condition most commonly affects two areas of your spine:

Lower back (lumbar spinal stenosis): Your lumbar spine consists of five bones (vertebrae) in your lower back. Your lumbar vertebrae, known as L1 to L5, are the largest of your entire spine.

Neck (cervical spinal stenosis): Your cervical spine consists of seven vertebrae in your neck. These vertebrae are labeled C1 to C7.

Your middle back (thoracic spine) can also have spinal stenosis, but this is rare.

Who Gets Spinal Stenosis?

Anyone can get spinal stenosis; however, the chances of developing the disorder increase with age. Degenerative spinal changes affect up to 95% of people by the age of 50. Spinal stenosis is one of those changes. For people over 65 undergoing spine surgery, lumbar spinal stenosis is the most common diagnosis. Spinal stenosis also can be present in younger people who are born with a narrow spinal canal or who have an injury to the spine.

Causes and Risk Factors

What causes spinal stenosis?

Spinal stenosis has several causes. Many different changes or injuries in your spine can cause a narrowing of your spinal canal. The causes are split into two main groups:

Acquired (developing after birth).

Congenital (from birth).

Acquired spinal stenosis is more common. It usually happens from "wear and tear" changes that naturally occur in your spine as you age. Only 9% of cases result from congenital causes.

Acquired causes of spinal stenosis

Acquired spinal stenosis means you develop it later in life (after birth) — most commonly after the age of 50. These cases usually happen from an injury or changes in your spine that occur as you age (degenerative changes).

Causes of acquired spinal stenosis include:

Bone overgrowth: Osteoarthritis is the "wear and tear" condition that breaks down the cartilage in your joints, including your spine. Cartilage is the protective covering of joints. As your cartilage wears away, your bones begin to rub against each other. Your body responds by growing new bone. Bone spurs, or an overgrowth of bone, commonly form. Bone spurs on your vertebrae extend into your spinal canal, narrowing the space and pinching nerves in your spine. Paget's disease of the bone can also cause an overgrowth of bone in your spine.

Bulging or herniated disks: Between each vertebra is a flat, round cushioning pad (vertebral disk) that acts as a shock absorber. As you age, the disks can dry out and flatten. Cracking in the outer edge of the disks can cause the gel-like center to break through. The bulging disk then presses on the nerves near the disk.

Thickened ligaments: Ligaments are the fiber bands that hold your spine together. Arthritis can cause ligaments to thicken over time and bulge into your spinal canal.

Spinal fractures and injuries: Broken or dislocated bones in your vertebrae or near your spine can narrow your canal space. Inflammation from injuries near your spine can also cause issues.

Spinal cysts or tumors: Growths within your spinal cord or between your spinal cord and vertebrae can narrow your spinal canal.

Congenital causes of spinal stenosis

Congenital spinal stenosis affects babies and children. It can happen due to:

Issues with spine formation during fetal development.

Genetic (inherited) conditions that affect bone growth. These are due to genetic mutations (changes).

Some congenital causes of spinal stenosis include:

Achondroplasia: A bone growth disorder that results in dwarfism due to a genetic mutation.

Spinal dysraphism: When the spine, spinal cord or nerve roots don't form properly during fetal development. Spina bifida and other neural tube defects are examples.

Congenital kyphosis: When your child's spine curves outward more than it should. As a result, their upper back looks overly rounded. This happens due to an issue with fetal spine development.

Congenital short pedicles: When your baby is born with vertebrae pedicles (the bony "sides" of the spinal canal) that are shorter in length. This decreases their spinal canal size.

Osteopetrosis: A rare genetic condition that causes your child's bones to grow abnormally and become overly dense.

Morquio syndrome: A rare genetic condition that affects your child's bones, spine and other body systems.

Hereditary multiple exostoses (diaphyseal aclasis): A rare genetic condition that causes several small bone growths (protrusions). They can grow on your child's vertebrae and affect their spinal canal.

Symptoms and Diagnosis

Symptoms of spinal stenosis may develop when the spaces within the spine narrow, most often in the lower back and neck. The narrowing creates pressure on the spine and related structures, causing symptoms. For most people, symptoms develop and progress slowly over a period of time, and some people may not have any symptoms.

The symptoms you experience depend on the location of the narrowing in your spine. Symptoms of spinal stenosis in the lower back can include:

Pain in the lower back.

Burning pain or ache that radiates down the buttocks and into the legs, that typically worsens with standing or walking and gets better with leaning forward (flexion).

Numbness, tingling, or cramping in the legs and feet. These may become more pronounced during standing or walking.

Weakness in the legs and feet.

Symptoms of spinal stenosis in the neck may include:

Neck pain.

Numbness or tingling that radiates down the arms into the hands.

Weakness in a hand, arm, or fingers.

Walking, standing, or extending the lumbar area of the spine can cause symptoms to worsen. Sitting or flexing the lower back or neck may relieve symptoms. The flexed position "opens up" the spinal column, enlarging the spaces between vertebrae at the back of the spine.

People with more severe stenosis also may have problems with:

Bowel function.

Bladder function.

Sexual function.

Diagnosis

How is spinal stenosis diagnosed?

Your healthcare provider will review your medical history, ask about your symptoms and do a physical exam. Your provider may feel your spine, pressing on different areas to see if it causes pain. They'll likely ask you to bend in different directions to see if certain spine positions bring on symptoms.

You'll also have imaging tests so your provider can "see" your spine and determine the exact location, type and extent of the problem. These tests may include:

Spine X-ray: X-rays use a small amount of radiation and can show changes in bone structure. For example, they can show a loss of disk height or bone spurs.

MRI: Magnetic resonance imaging (MRI) uses radio waves and a powerful magnet to create cross-sectional images of your spine. MRI provides detailed images of your nerves, disks and spinal cord. It can reveal any tumors as well.

CT scan or CT myelogram: A computed tomography (CT) scan is a combination of X-rays that creates cross-sectional images of your spine. A CT myelogram uses a contrast dye so your provider can more clearly see your spinal cord and nerves.

Treatment strategies

Doctors treat spinal stenosis with different options such as nonsurgical treatments, medications, and surgical treatments.

Nonsurgical Treatments

Physical therapy to maintain motion of the spine, strengthen abdominal and back muscles, and build endurance, all of which help stabilize the spine. You may be encouraged to try slowly progressive aerobic activity, such as swimming or using exercise bicycles. In addition, your physical therapist or health care provider may recommend home exercises.

A brace to provide some support and help you regain mobility. This approach is sometimes used for people with weak abdominal muscles or older patients with age-related changes at several levels of the spine.

Complementary and alternative treatments that may help relieve pain. Some examples include:

Manipulation of the spine and nearby tissues. Professionals use their hands to adjust and massage the spine and muscles.

Acupuncture, which is a Chinese practice that uses thin needles that may relieve pain in some patients.

How you can help to improve your own symptoms

Maintain activity as much as you can. Try to gradually increase the distance you walk if you can.

Try to lose weight if you are overweight.

Medications

Your doctor may prescribe one or more of the following medications to help manage the pain and inflammation caused by spinal stenosis:

Anti–inflammatory medications to help relieve inflammation and pain.

Over-the-counter pain relievers taken by mouth or applied to the skin.

Pain relief. Using over-the-counter medication such as paracetamol or ibuprofen may be sufficient. Other medicines prescribed by your doctor can be used if over-the-counter medicines do not provide enough pain relief. Some medicines can be used specifically to help the nerve pain in your legs - for example, amitriptyline, gabapentin or pregabalin.

Anti-inflammatory or numbing injections for pain that radiates or travels due to nerve compression or irritation.

Surgical Treatments

If, after trying nonsurgical treatments and medications, you still have symptoms, your doctor may recommend meeting with a surgeon to talk about surgery. However, doctors may recommend surgery right away if you have numbness or weakness that interferes with walking, impaired bowel or bladder function, or other neurological involvement.

The decision to have surgery depends on:

How nonsurgical treatments have helped your symptoms.

The amount of pain you feel.

Other diseases and conditions you may have.

Your overall health.

Whether your specific spinal anatomy is amenable to surgery.

However, not everyone is a candidate for surgery, even if symptoms persist. In addition, your surgeon will review the risks and possible benefits of the surgery or procedure.

Surgeons can relieve pressure on the spinal cord and nerves, and restore spine alignment and health by performing surgery. Possible surgeries include:

Laminectomy is a surgery that doctors perform to treat spinal stenosis by removing the bony spurs and the bone walls of the vertebrae. This helps to open up the spinal column and remove the pressure on the nerves. Doctors may perform a discectomy during a laminectomy. A discectomy involves removing part of the herniated disk to relieve pressure on the spinal cord or nerve root. A facetectomy involves removing part or all of a facet joint to relieve pressure.

Spinal fusion is a surgery that helps treat age-related changes to the spine and spondylolisthesis by joining two or more vertebrae in the spine that have slipped from their normal position. During this procedure, the surgeon may remove the disk between the vertebrae and uses bone grafts or metal devices to secure bones together.

Minimally invasive surgery is a type of surgery that uses smaller incisions than standard surgery. Minimally invasive surgery may cause less scarring and damage to nearby muscles and other tissues. It can lead to less pain and faster recovery after surgery.

Removing and repairing the areas of spine that are creating pressure usually helps decrease symptoms. Most people have less leg pain and can walk better after surgery. However, if nerves were badly damaged before surgery, there may be some remaining pain or numbness or no improvement. Also, the degenerative process may continue, and pain or limitation of activity may reappear after surgery.

PART II: Role of Diet in Managing Spinal Stenosis Symptoms

While there are effective conventional and natural treatments that help manage spinal stenosis, eating a healthy diet can also help relieve many symptoms associated with this spine condition. If you are suffering from spinal stenosis, be sure to incorporate the following into your diet…

Healthy Proteins such as lean meats, fish, eggs, and tofu are great selections as they play an important role in healing and also repairing and maintaining bone and cartilage.

Calcium is a mineral that plays an important role in maintaining strong bones as you age. Just a few great sources of calcium include wild caught salmon, almonds, dairy products, and green leafy vegetables.

Magnesium is another mineral that is very beneficial for maintaining bone density and muscle strength. Be sure to consume magnesium rich foods such as bananas, avocados, almonds, spinach, brown rice, and broccoli!

Vitamin D3 is great for bone health because it helps you to absorb calcium! Great sources of Vitamin D3 include egg yolks, cheese, fatty fish such as tuna, mackerel, and salmon, as well as foods fortified with Vitamin D such as orange juice, soy milk, cereal, and some dairy products.

Fluids

Drinking adequate fluids will help your spinal discs stay hydrated. These discs provide cushioning between your vertebrae and facilitate movement in your spinal joints. Hydration benefits your discs by contributing to their fluid content. To keep up your fluid intake, drink water and other calorie-free or low-calorie beverages throughout the day. Limit or eliminate caffeinated drinks and alcohol, which may leave you dehydrated.

Foods to Include and Avoid in a Spinal Stenosis Diet

Certain foods are packed with what your back needs in order to remain healthy and strong. So good back health can start with making the right food choices.

Avoiding bad foods is one way to increase health. Choosing the right ones is the best way to go. Foods rich in essential nutrients for spinal health include:

Plant-Based Proteins

The proteins you get from certain plants are great for your spine health. These proteins are different than the ones found in meat.

Stick to plant-based proteins as much as possible. Animal-based proteins can lead to inflammation.

Instead, get your protein from foods like chia seeds, lentils, and beans. Not only do they provide protein, they pack a nutritional punch in other ways, too. You'll get a variety of helpful antioxidants, fiber, vitamins, and minerals as well.

If you'd still like to get some animal-based protein in your diet, go for lean picks. This means choosing chicken and fish over beef and pork.

Vegetables

Vegetables are good for you in general, so make sure you get a lot of them each day to improve your overall health. While healthy all around, veggies are also great for fighting back issues.

Certain vegetables contain properties that will help fight spinal issues.

Kale, broccoli, and spinach work well against inflammation. Each of these vegetables also contains nutrients that will help strengthen your spine. As the literal backbone of your body's skeletal system, your spine can use all the nutritional help it can get.

As a rule of thumb, veggies with strong natural pigments are best.

Salmon

If you're not opposed to seafood, add some salmon to your diet regularly. Salmon is a great source of lean protein, as well as well as another helpful nutrient: omega-3 fatty acids.

Omega-3 fatty acids promote bone and tissue health. They also fight against inflammation, just like those leafy green vegetables mentioned above.

Luckily, salmon is versatile and tasty when prepared the right way. There are plenty of fantastic salmon dishes for you to try. They'll spice up your menu and benefit your back at the same time.

Dairy Products

Calcium is super important for maintaining and improving bone health. The easiest way to get extra calcium in your diet without taking a supplement? Increase your dairy intake.

Don't choose just any dairy products, though. Specifically, go for the ones that are high in calcium. Cheese, milk, and yogurt all fall into this category.

Like with many other food groups, though, you can overdo it with dairy. Don't binge on your favorite cheese with the excuse of needing the extra calcium.

Be smart about how you eat dairy products so you don't get too much fat or cholesterol in your diet.

Calcium can be found in other foods, too. Among them are those leafy green vegetables we've already talked about.

Herbs and Spices

Many herbs and spices are great for promoting spinal health. Turmeric, a spice commonly used in Indian cuisine, including curry dishes, helps fix damaged tissue.

There are herbs that fight inflammation as well. These include cinnamon, rosemary, basil, and ginger.

Add these and other healthy spices and herbs to your recipes throughout the day. Or use them to create a healthy, delicious herbal tea. Herbal teas help strengthen your immune system, reduce inflammation, and taste great at the same time.

Fruits

Just like vegetables, you should go for the highly-pigmented types here. And like dairy, you don't want to overdo it. Remember, fruit is sugar, so eating too much can be more of a detriment to your health than a benefit.

While you need to be responsible when eating fruits, they have many health benefits.

Berries are particularly great for your spinal health. They're packed with antioxidants and nutrients that will help your spine get and stay healthy.

So add those berries to breakfasts, dinners, lunches, you name it. You can even use them as dessert.

Avocados

Whether you're a fan of avocados or not, they're great for your spine. They're full of healthy fats that your body needs as well as fiber and potassium. These things make avocados great for your health overall.

Whether it's good fat or not, avocados are fatty foods, so make sure you don't overdo it.

If you don't like avocados, try using them in ways you haven't before. In recent years tons of recipes have emerged for avocado toast, addition to a smoothie and other tasty meals. You don't have to limit yourself to a plain slice with a salad or a guacamole dip.

One of the greatest things about avocados? They help to reduce back pain.

Foods to Limit or Avoid to Reduce Inflammation and Pain

Limiting certain foods in your diet can help manage spinal stenosis. Here's what to watch out for:

Foods to Limit:

Processed Foods: They're often packed with unhealthy fats, sugars, and additives that can fuel inflammation.

Saturated and Trans Fats: These lurk in fried foods, baked goods, and processed snacks, ramping up inflammation levels.

Sugary Treats: Think sodas, candies, and desserts; they not only add to inflammation but also to your waistline.

Refined Carbs: Foods like white bread, rice, and pasta can cause blood sugar spikes, aggravating inflammation.

Red Meat: Too much beef and pork can amp up inflammation. Instead, lean towards leaner proteins like poultry, fish, or plant-based options.

Excess Salt: A high-sodium diet can cause water retention and worsen inflammation. Try flavoring with herbs and spices instead.

Alcohol: Overindulging can up inflammation and mess with bone health. Moderation or skipping it altogether is key.

Foods to Avoid:

Trans Fats: Found in partially hydrogenated oils, these fats spell trouble and should be cut out entirely.

Processed Meats: Bacon, sausage, and deli meats are loaded with additives that can worsen inflammation.

High-Glycemic Foods: Foods like sugary cereals, pastries, and white potatoes can spike blood sugar and inflammation.

Sugary Drinks: Sodas, energy drinks, and sweetened teas offer no nutritional value and only serve to inflame.

Too Much Caffeine: While a little is okay, too much can mess with calcium absorption and bone health.

Artificial Sweeteners: Some studies hint they might worsen inflammation; best to steer clear if possible.

PART III: Lifestyle Modifications to Support Spinal Stenosis Management

Many people can manage their symptoms and lead an active life despite this condition, there are some tips that can help.

1. Take a dip

Exercise can help build muscles in the legs, abdomen and back. Stronger muscles can support the spine and take some pressure off the pinched nerves.

Any exercise you enjoy can help. But experts recommend water exercise if you can get to a pool.

Swimming and other aquatic activities are great for spinal stenosis because you use the buoyancy of water to your advantage. Water workouts are easier on the spine and all the joints. At the same time, the resistance in the water helps you strengthen your muscles.

2. Lean into your activity

In the absence of a pool, you have other exercise options. Exercises that allow you to lean forward slightly, including:

Biking or using a stationary bike.

Walking up a flight of stairs.

Using a stage climbing machine.

Using a treadmill with an incline.

Many people find that leaning forward offers them relief from spinal pressure because it opens up the spine a little bit.

However, if you're in too much pain to exercise, it is not recommended to push through it alone. If you're skipping activities or you can't function normally, make an appointment with your doctor, there are plenty of treatment options that could help you.

3. Work on weight loss

Excess weight can worsen the pain of spinal stenosis. Extra body weight puts additional pressure on the spine, while losing weight can bring relief.

If you're getting more active with the tips mentioned above, you may already have this covered. Exercise is a great way to burn calories and work toward a healthy weight.

But also watch your diet for maximum weight loss success. Eating too many calories could undo the calorie burning you accomplished on that bike ride.

4. Try turmeric

Turmeric is a plant related to ginger, and people have used it for thousands of years. It's a flavorful spice for cooking, but you can also take it as a supplement. Turmeric has some promising evidence of pain relief.

We don't have solid proof that turmeric works for spinal stenosis pain. However, some studies show that it could help relieve arthritis pain. And arthritis is a common trigger of spinal stenosis.

Therefore, turmeric may be worth a try, along with exercise and weight loss. It could interact with certain medicines, however, so ask your doctor first.

5. **Give PT a chance**

Physical therapy (PT) is completely noninvasive and highly effective.

Physical therapy is the hallmark of treatment for spinal stenosis. The goal is to condition the muscles to decrease pressure on the areas of pain.

During a PT appointment, a licensed physical therapist guides you through strengthening or stretching exercises. The therapist customizes these exercises for your areas of pain, fitness level and body type.

Seems simple, right? So can you just look up online videos for spinal stenosis exercises? You can do that, but you won't get the same results. A physical therapist is an expert in the musculoskeletal system. And having an expert will always get you the best outcome.

If you go this route, you may find that the exercises are challenging. PT requires time and effort, but the benefit comes with the effort you put in.

PART IV 4: RECIPES AND MEAL IDEAS FOR SPINAL STENOSIS

BREAKFAST RECIPES FOR SPINAL STENOSIS

Spicy Moroccan eggs

Ingredients

- 2 tsp rapeseed oil

- 1 large onion, halved and thinly sliced

- 3 garlic cloves, sliced

- 1 tbsp rose harissa

- 1 tsp ground coriander

- 150ml vegetable stock

- 400g can chickpea

- 2 x 400g cans cherry tomatoes

- 2 courgettes, finely diced

- 200g bag baby spinach

- 4 tbsp chopped coriander

- 4 large eggs

Method

- STAGE 1

Heat the oil in a large, deep frying pan, and fry the onion and garlic for about 8 mins, stirring every now and then, until starting to turn golden. Add the harissa and ground coriander, stir well, then pour in the stock and chickpeas with their liquid. Cover and simmer for 5 mins, then mash about one-third of the chickpeas to thicken the stock a little.

• STAGE 2

Tip the tomatoes and courgettes into the pan, and cook gently for 10 mins until the courgettes are tender. Fold in the spinach so that it wilts into the pan.

• STAGE 3

Stir in the chopped coriander, then make 4 hollows in the mixture and break in the eggs. Cover and cook for 2 mins, then take off the heat and allow to settle for 2 mins before serving.

Staffordshire oatcakes with mushrooms

Ingredients

For the oatcakes

• 85g porridge oats

• 85g plain wholemeal flour

• ½ tsp dried yeast

For the topping

• 4 tsp rapeseed oil, plus a little for frying

• 320g button mushrooms, sliced

• 4 tomatoes, each cut into 8 wedges

• 4 tbsp milled seeds with flax and chia

• 4 tbsp tahini

• A few coriander sprigs, chopped

Method

• STAGE 1

For the oatcakes, tip the oats and 350ml water into a bowl and blitz with a stick blender until smooth (alternatively you can use a food processor or liquidizer). Stir in the flour and yeast, cover and leave in the fridge overnight, or leave at room temperature for 2-3 hrs until bubbles appear.

• STAGE 2

Use kitchen paper to rub ½ tsp oil round a non-stick frying pan, then heat. Ladle in a quarter of the batter and swirl the pan to cover the base (the oatcakes should be a few millimeters thick, like a crêpe). Cook for 2 mins, then turn and cook for 2 mins more until golden. Make four oatcakes in the same way. If you're following our Healthy Diet Plan, chill two for another day. Will keep, covered in the fridge, for two days.

• STAGE 3

To make the topping for two oatcakes, heat 2 tsp oil in a non-stick pan, add 160g mushrooms and fry for 2-3 mins, stirring until softened. Stir in 2 tomatoes, then add 2 tbsp ground seeds and cook for 2 mins more. Reheat the oatcakes in a dry frying pan or the microwave if necessary, then spread each one with 1 tbsp tahini, the mushroom mixture and scatter with a little coriander before serving. On the second day, repeat stage 3 with the remaining Ingredients.

Pancakes for one

Ingredients

• 1 large egg

• 40g plain flour

* ½ tsp baking powder

* 45ml milk (dairy, nut or oat based)

* 1 tsp butter

* ½ tbsp oil

* maple syrup or honey and berries, to serve (optional)

Method

* STAGE 1

Separate the egg, putting the white and yolk in separate bowls. Mix the egg yolk with the flour, baking powder and milk to make a smooth paste.

* STAGE 2

Beat the egg white and a pinch of salt with an electric whisk (or by hand) until fluffy and holding its shape. Gently fold the egg white into the yolk mixture. Be extra careful not to knock any of the air out.

• STAGE 3

Heat the butter and oil in a non-stick frying pan. Dollop a third of the mixture into the pan and cook on each side for 1-2 mins or until golden brown. Repeat with the remaining mixture to make three pancakes. Drizzle over some maple syrup or honey and serve with berries, if you like.

Overnight oats with apricots & yogurt

Ingredients

For the oats

• 200g oats

• 50g chia seeds

• 1 tbsp vanilla extract

• 550ml almond milk, or cow's milk (if non-vegan)

For the apricots

• 1 tsp rapeseed oil

• 320g pack fresh apricots, stoned and quartered

• 400g pot fortified oat or plain bio yogurt

• 4 tsp sunflower seeds

Method

• STAGE 1

Mix the oats and chia in a bowl with the vanilla and almond milk. Cover and chill overnight.

• STAGE 2

Heat the oil in a small non-stick pan. Add the apricots in a single layer, then cover the pan and cook over a low heat for 5 mins, until softened. Stir well and cook a few minutes more if needed – they will cook a little more in the residual heat as they cool. Cover and keep chilled until needed.

• STAGE 3

The next day, stir the yogurt into the oats and spoon into tumblers, small jars or small bowls. Top with the cooked apricots and sunflower seeds. Will keep covered and chilled for up to four days.

Green fritters

Ingredients

• 140g courgettes, grated

• 3 medium eggs

• 85g broccoli florets, finely chopped

• small pack dill, roughly chopped

• 3 tbsp gluten-free flour or rice flour

• 2 tbsp sunflower oil, for frying

Method

• STAGE 1

Squeeze the courgettes between your hands to remove any excess moisture, or tip onto a clean tea towel and twist it to squeeze out the moisture.

• STAGE 2

Beat the eggs in a bowl, add the broccoli, courgettes and most of the dill, and mix together. Add the flour, mix again and season.

• STAGE 3

Heat the oil in a non-stick frying pan. Put a large serving spoon of the mixture in the pan, then add 2 more spoonfuls so you have 3 fritters. Leave for 3-4 mins on a medium heat until golden brown on one side and solid enough for you to flip over, then flip over and leave to go golden on the other side. Repeat to make 3 more fritters (there is no need to add any more oil to the pan after the first batch). Scatter with the remaining dill to serve.

Porridge with blueberry compote

Ingredients

• 6 tbsp porridge oats

• just under ½ x 200ml tub 0% fat Greek-style yogurt

• ½ x 350g pack frozen blueberries

• 1 tsp honey (optional)

Method

• STAGE 1

Put the oats in a non-stick pan with 400ml water and cook over the heat, stirring occasionally for about 2 minutes until thickened. Remove from the heat and add a third of the yogurt.

• STAGE 2

Meanwhile, tip the blueberries into a pan with 1 tbsp water and the honey if using and gently poach until the blueberries have thawed and they are tender, but still holding their shape.

• STAGE 3

Spoon the porridge into bowls, top with the remaining yogurt and spoon over the blueberries.

Vegan tomato & mushroom pancakes

Ingredients

140g white self-raising flour

1 tsp soya flour

400ml soya milk

vegetable oil, for frying

For the topping

2 tbsp vegetable oil

250g button mushrooms

250g cherry tomatoes, halved

2 tbsp soya cream or soya milk

large handful pine nuts

snipped chives, to serve

Directions

STAGE 1

Sift the flours and a pinch of salt into a blender. Add the soya milk and blend to make a smooth batter.

STAGE 2

Heat a little oil in a medium non-stick frying pan until very hot. Pour about 3 tbsp of the batter into the pan and cook over a medium heat until bubbles appear on the surface of the pancake. Flip the pancake over with a palette knife and cook the other side until golden brown. Repeat with the remaining batter, keeping the cooked pancakes warm as you go. You will make about 8.

STAGE 3

For the topping, heat the oil in a frying pan. Cook the mushrooms until tender, add the tomatoes and cook for a couple of mins. Pour in the soya cream or milk and pine nuts, then gently cook until combined. Divide the pancakes between 2 plates, then spoon over the tomatoes and mushrooms. Scatter with chives.

Crumpets

Ingredients

2½ tsp dried yeast

240ml warm milk

2 tbsp unsalted butter, melted

2tsp sea salt

2tsp caster sugar

470g plain flour

½ tsp baking powder dissolved in 60ml warm water

vegetable oil, to grease

butter or cheese, to serve

Directions

STAGE 1

Stir together the yeast and 240ml warm water in a bowl and leave to stand for 5-10 mins. Add the warm milk, butter, salt and sugar, then tip in the flour and stir until smooth. Leave to stand for 30 mins.

STAGE 2

Dissolve the baking powder in a little water, then leave to rise for 20-30 mins.

STAGE 3

Oil a heavy-based frying pan with a little vegetable oil and heat over medium-low heat. Lightly oil four 9cm crumpet rings. Spoon batter into the rings so it comes halfway up the sides. Reduce heat to low, cover with a lid, or an upturned deep frying pan to give the crumpets space to rise. Cook until the tops look dry, about 10-12 mins.

STAGE 4

Flip them over and cook for 5 mins until golden and firm. Repeat with the remaining batter. Serve toasted with butter or topped with cheese, melted under the grill.

Carrot & pecan muffins

Ingredients

2 x 400g can cannellini beans in water, drained

2 tsp ground cinnamon

100g porridge oats

4 large eggs

2 tbsp rapeseed oil

4 tbsp maple syrup

2 tsp vanilla extract

zest 1 large orange

170g carrot, coarsely grated

100g raisins

80g pecan halves, 12 reserved, the rest roughly chopped

2 tsp baking powder

Directions

STAGE 1

Heat oven to 180C/160C fan/gas 4 and line a 12-hole muffin tin with paper cases. Tip the beans into a bowl and add the cinnamon, oats, eggs, oil, maple syrup, vanilla extract and orange zest. Blitz with a hand blender until really smooth – the beans and oats should be ground down as much as possible.

STAGE 2

Stir in the carrot, raisins, chopped pecans and baking powder, and mix well. Spoon into the muffin cases – use a large ice cream scoop if you have one, to get nice even muffins.

STAGE 3

Top each muffin with a reserved pecan and bake for 20 mins until set and light brown. Cool on a wire rack. Will keep in the fridge for a few days, or freeze for 6 weeks; thaw at room temperature.

Cinnamon roll pancakes

Ingredients

145g self-raising flour

1 tsp baking powder

1 tbsp golden caster sugar

1 tsp cinnamon

2 eggs

40g butter, melted

140ml milk

3 tbsp light brown soft sugar

1 tbsp maple syrup, plus extra to serve (optional)

1 tbsp vegetable oil

6 tbsp toffee or caramel yogurt, to serve (optional)

Directions

STAGE 1

Weigh the flour in a large jug or bowl. Add the baking powder, caster sugar, ½ tsp cinnamon and a generous pinch of salt. Whisk to combine. Crack in the eggs, add ½ the butter and all the milk, then whisk to a smooth batter. Will keep in the fridge overnight.

STAGE 2

Stir the rest of the cinnamon, the light brown sugar and the maple syrup into the remaining melted butter. Add 3 tbsp of the pancake mixture and mix. Transfer to a squeezy bottle fitted with a small nozzle or a piping bag.

STAGE 3

When you're ready to cook, pour a little oil in your largest frying pan, and wipe out any excess with some kitchen paper. Keeping the pan over a low-medium heat, spoon 2-3 tbsp mounds into the pan for each pancake, leaving space for them to expand as they cook. You should get three or four in at a time. Use the cinnamon mixture in your bottle or piping bag to pipe swirls on top of each pancake. When the pancakes start to set around the edges and you see bubbles appear on top, carefully flip and cook for another 2-3 mins until golden and cooked through. Keep warm in a low oven while you continue cooking the rest of the batter.

STAGE 4

Serve the pancakes with yogurt and extra maple syrup, if you like.

Creamy yogurt porridge with apple & raisin compote

Ingredients

For the compote

2 apples, peeled and thickly sliced

25g raisin

150ml orange juice

small handful of sunflower seeds

For the porridge

6 tbsp (50g) porridge oat

300g pot 0% fat probiotic plain yogurt

Directions

STAGE 1

For the apple topping: Poach apples in a covered pan with raisins and orange juice for 8-10 mins until the apple is tender. Mash a little of the apple to thicken the juice. Can be made ahead and chilled for up to 1 week. Serve warm or cold on the porridge with sunflower seeds.

STAGE 2

For the porridge: Tip 400ml water into a small non-stick pan and stir in porridge oats. Cook over a low heat until bubbling and thickened. (To make in a microwave, use a deep container to prevent spillage as the mixture will rise up as it cooks, and cook for 3 mins on High.) Stir in yogurt – or swirl in half and top with the rest.

Ultimate Seville orange marmalade

Ingredients

1.3kg Seville orange

2 lemons, juice only

2.6kg preserving or granulated sugar

Directions

STAGE 1

Put the whole oranges and lemon juice in a large
preserving pan and cover with 2 litres/4 pints water -
if it does not cover the fruit, use a smaller pan. If
necessary weight the oranges with a heat-proof plate
to keep them submerged. Bring to the boil, cover and
simmer very gently for around 2 hours, or until the
peel can be easily pierced with a fork.

STAGE 2

Warm half the sugar in a very low oven. Pour off the
cooking water from the oranges into a jug and tip the
oranges into a bowl. Return cooking liquid to the

pan. Allow oranges to cool until they are easy to handle, then cut in half. Scoop out all the pips and pith and add to the reserved orange liquid in the pan. Bring to the boil for 6 minutes, then strain this liquid through a sieve into a bowl and press the pulp through with a wooden spoon - it is high in pectin so gives marmalade a good set.

STAGE 3

Pour half this liquid into a preserving pan. Cut the peel, with a sharp knife, into fine shreds. Add half the peel to the liquid in the preserving pan with the warm sugar. Stir over a low heat until all the sugar has dissolved, for about 10 minutes, then bring to the boil and bubble rapidly for 15- 25 minutes until setting point is reached.

STAGE 4

Take pan off the heat and skim any scum from the surface. (To dissolve any excess scum, drop a small knob of butter on to the surface, and gently stir.)

Leave the marmalade to stand in the pan for 20 minutes to cool a little and allow the peel to settle; then pot in sterilised jars, seal and label. Repeat from stage 3 for second batch, warming the other half of the sugar first.

Date & buckwheat granola with pecans & seeds

Ingredients

For the granola

85g buckwheat

4 medjool dates, stoned

1 tsp ground cinnamon

100g traditional oats

2 tsp rapeseed oil

25g sunflower seeds

25g pumpkin seeds

25g flaked almonds

50g pecan nuts, roughly broken into halves

50g sultanas (without added oil)

For the yogurt & fruit (to serve 2)

2 x 150ml pots low-fat bio natural yogurt

2 ripe nectarines or peaches, stoned and sliced

Directions

STAGE 1

Soak the buckwheat overnight in cold water. The next day, drain and rinse the buckwheat. Put the dates in a pan with 300ml water and the cinnamon, and blitz with a stick blender until completely smooth. Add the buckwheat, bring to the boil and cook, uncovered, for 5 mins until pulpy. Meanwhile, heat oven to 150C/130C fan/gas 2 and line two large baking trays with baking parchment.

STAGE 2

Stir the oats and oil into the date and buckwheat mixture, then spoon small clusters of the mixture onto the baking trays. Bake for 15 mins, then carefully scrape the clusters from the parchment if they have stuck and turn before spreading out again. Return to the oven for another 15 mins, turning frequently, until firm and golden.

STAGE 3

When the mix is dry enough, tip into a bowl, mix in the seeds and nuts with the sultanas and toss well. When cool, serve each person a generous handful with yogurt and fruit, and pack the excess into an airtight container. Will keep for a week. On other

days you can vary the fruit or serve with milk or a
dairy-free alternative instead of the yogurt.

Eggs benedict

Ingredients

3 tbsp white wine vinegar

4 eggs

2 toasting muffins

4 parma ham

For the hollandaise sauce

125g butter

2 egg yolks

½ tsp white wine vinegar or tarragon vinegar

squeeze of lemon juice

pinch of cayenne pepper

Directions

To prepare:

STAGE 1

Bring a deep saucepan of water to the boil (at least 2 litres) and add 3 tbsp white wine vinegar. Lower the heat down to a gentle simmer.

STAGE 2

Break the eggs into four separate coffee cups or ramekins. Split the muffins, toast them for a few minutes either side and warm some plates.

To make the hollandaise:

STAGE 1

Melt the butter in a saucepan and skim any white solids from the surface. Keep the butter warm.

STAGE 2

Put the egg yolks, white wine or tarragon vinegar, a pinch of salt and a splash of ice-cold water in a metal or glass bowl that will fit over a small pan. Whisk for a few minutes, then put the bowl over a pan of barely simmering water and whisk continuously until pale and thick, about 3-5 mins.

STAGE 3

Remove from the heat and slowly whisk in the melted butter bit by bit until it's all incorporated and you have a creamy hollandaise. (If it gets too thick, add a splash of water.) Season with a squeeze of lemon juice and a little cayenne pepper. Keep warm until needed.

To make the eggs benedict:

STAGE 1

Swirl the simmering vinegared water briskly to form a vortex and slide in an egg. It will curl round and set to a neat round shape. Cook for 2-3 mins, then remove with a slotted spoon.

STAGE 2

Repeat with the other eggs, one at a time, re-swirling the water as you slide in the eggs. Spread some sauce on each muffin, scrunch a slice of ham on top, then top with an egg. Spoon over the remaining hollandaise and serve at once.

Butternut & cinnamon oats

Ingredients

120g porridge oats

80g raisins

2 tsp ground cinnamon, plus a sprinkling to serve

large chunk butternut squash, peeled and coarsely grated (approx 320g grated weight)

2 x 150ml pots bio yogurt

25g walnuts roughly broken

milk, to serve (optional)

Directions

STAGE 1

Tip the oats, raisins and cinnamon into a large bowl and pour over 1 litre cold water. Cover the bowl and leave to soak overnight.

STAGE 2

The next morning, tip the contents into a large saucepan and stir in the grated squash. Cook for about 8-10 mins over a medium heat, stirring frequently, until the oats are cooked and the squash is soft. Add a little more water if it's too thick.

STAGE 3

Put half of the mixture in the fridge for the next day. Spoon the remainder into bowls, top each portion with 1 pot yogurt and half the nuts. Dust with cinnamon, then serve with a splash of milk.

LUNCH RECIPES FOR SPINAL STENOSIS

Spicy avocado wraps

Ingredients

0.5 x 300g pack mycoprotein chicken-style pieces (or similar vegetarian product), sliced at an angle

generous squeeze juice 0.5 lime

½ tsp mild chilli powder

1 garlic clove, chopped

1 tsp olive oil

2 seeded wraps

1 avocado, halved and stoned

1 roasted red pepper, from a jar

few sprigs coriander, chopped

Directions

STAGE 1

Mix the vegetarian, chicken-style pieces with the lime juice, chilli powder and garlic.

STAGE 2

Heat the oil in a non-stick frying pan then fry the pieces for a couple of mins, while you warm the wraps following the pack instructions or if you have a gas hob, heat them over the flame to slightly char them. Do not let them dry out or they are difficult to roll.

STAGE 3

Squash half an avocado onto each wrap, add the peppers to the pan to warm them through then pile onto the wraps with the chicken-style pieces, and sprinkle over the coriander. Roll up, cut in half and eat with your fingers.

Lemon roast vegetables with yogurt tahini & pomegranate

Ingredients

1 red pepper, deseeded and chopped

1 aubergine, diced

1 red onion, halved and thinly sliced

1 unwaxed lemon, 1/4 finely chopped (skin and all), the rest juiced

1 tbsp rapeseed oil, plus extra to drizzle (optional)

400g can chickpeas in water, drained

1 garlic clove

2 tbsp tahini

3 tbsp natural bio yogurt

seeds from ½ a pomegranate

⅓ small pack parsley or coriander, chopped

Directions

STAGE 1

Heat oven to 240C/220C fan/gas 7. Put the vegetables and chopped lemon in a large flameproof roasting tin and drizzle with 1 tbsp oil. Massage into the veg so they are all well coated, then put the tin on the hob and fry, stirring, for 5 mins until starting to char. Stir in two handfuls of the chickpeas, and roast in the oven for 15 mins.

STAGE 2

Put the rest of the chickpeas in a bowl with the garlic, tahini, yogurt, lemon juice and 3 tbsp water, and blitz with a stick blender until really smooth and thick.

STAGE 3

Spoon the yogurt tahini onto two plates and top with the roasted veg, pomegranate seeds and parsley. Season with black pepper and a drizzle of extra oil, if you like.

Ricotta, broccoli & lemon penne

Ingredients

200g wholemeal penne

1 leek, washed and sliced

200g broccoli, cut into small florets

1 tbsp rapeseed oil

1 red pepper, deseeded, quartered and sliced

1 tsp finely chopped rosemary

1 red chilli, deseeded and sliced

3 garlic cloves, sliced

1 lemon, zested and juiced

3 tbsp ricotta

Directions

STAGE 1

Boil the pasta with the leeks for 7 mins, then add the broccoli and boil for 5 mins more until just tender.

STAGE 2

Meanwhile, heat the oil and fry the pepper with the rosemary, chilli and garlic in a large non-stick pan for 5 mins until softened.

STAGE 3

Drain the pasta and veg, reserving a little water, then tip the pasta and veg into the pan. Add the lemon zest and juice, ricotta, and some pasta water. Pile into bowls.

Tuna, avocado & pea salad in Baby Gem lettuce wraps

Ingredients

1 ½ tbsp low-fat natural yogurt

85g canned tuna chunks (in spring water), drained

50g cooked and cooled rice (use leftover from Prawn, butternut & mango curry dinner if made - see 'goes well with', right)

85g frozen pea, cooked, then refreshed in cold water

½ red pepper, chopped

1 avocado, stoned, peeled and cut into chunks

zest and juice 1 lime

small pack coriander, chopped

1 large Baby Gem lettuce, or other crisp lettuce, such as cos

Directions

STAGE 1

Combine all the Ingredients except the lettuce in a bowl, season, then chill until ready to eat. Spoon the tuna mix on top of the lettuce leaves, wrap up and enjoy.

Penne with broccoli, lemon & anchovies

Ingredients

170g wholemeal penne

1 leek, washed and sliced

180g broccoli, cut into small florets

2 tsp oil from the anchovy can, plus 15g anchovies, chopped

1 red pepper, seeded, quartered and sliced

½ tsp finely chopped rosemary

1 red chilli, seeded and sliced

3 garlic cloves, sliced

½ lemon, zested and juiced

4 tbsp ricotta

2 tbsp sunflower seeds

Directions

STAGE 1

Boil the pasta with the sliced leek for 7 mins, then add the broccoli and boil for 5 mins until everything is just tender.

STAGE 2

Meanwhile, heat the oil from the anchovies and fry the red pepper with the rosemary, chilli and garlic in a large non-stick pan for 5 mins until softened.

STAGE 3

Drain the pasta, reserving a little water, then tip the pasta and veg into the pan and add the lemon juice and zest, anchovies and ricotta. Toss well over the heat, using the pasta water to moisten. Toss through the sunflower seeds and serve.

Balsamic lentil pies with vegetable mash

Ingredients

2 tbsp rapeseed oil, plus a drop extra

4 red onions, thinly sliced

200g puy lentils

2 tbsp finely chopped rosemary

1 tbsp vegetable bouillon powder

2 tbsp balsamic vinegar

350g peeled and diced celeriac

350g peeled and diced swede

350g peeled and diced potato

2 x 160g broccoli

2 x 160g spinach

50g vegetarian Italian-style hard cheese, finely grated

Directions

STAGE 1

Heat the oil in a large non-stick pan and fry the onions for 8 mins until softened and golden. Put a full kettle on to boil. Stir the lentils, rosemary, bouillon and balsamic vinegar into the onions, pour in 1 litre boiling water and simmer for 35-40 mins until the lentils are soft but still have some bite.

STAGE 2

Meanwhile, steam or boil the root veg for 25 mins and half the broccoli for 12-15 mins. Wilt half the spinach for 2 mins in a hot pan with a drop of oil.

STAGE 3

Mash the root veg with a hand blender or masher. Spoon the lentils into four individual pie dishes, top with the mash, then scatter over the cheese. While they're still hot, grill two pies to melt the cheese and serve with the cooked green veg. Chill the rest until needed. Will keep for three days in the fridge. To reheat the pies, bake in the oven at 180C/160C fan/gas 4 for 35 mins. Cook the rest of the green veg (as above) to serve alongside.

Chicken & lemon skewers

Ingredients

1 small pack mint, leaves picked

150g natural yogurt, plus extra to serve (optional)

1 lemon, zested and juiced

½ tsp ground cumin

½ tsp ground coriander

2cm piece ginger, grated

4 skinless chicken breasts, each cut into 6 pieces

4 wholemeal flatbreads or pittas

2 Little Gem lettuces, sliced

1 small red onion, sliced, to serve

pickled red cabbage, chilli sauce and hummus, to serve (all optional)

You will need

4 metal or wooden skewers

Directions

STAGE 1

Chop half the mint and put in a bowl with the yogurt, half the lemon juice, all the lemon zest, spices and ginger. Mix well and season with lots of black pepper and a pinch of salt. Add the chicken pieces, mix well and put in the fridge for 20-30 mins. Meanwhile, soak 4 large wooden skewers in water for at least 20 mins (or use metal ones).

STAGE 2

When you're ready to cook the chicken, heat your grill to a medium heat and line the grill tray with foil.

Thread the chicken onto the soaked wooden or metal skewers and grill for 15-20 mins, turning halfway through, until browned and cooked through.

STAGE 3

Warm the flatbreads under the grill for a couple of seconds, then serve them topped with the lettuce, chicken, red onion, remaining lemon juice and mint, and any optional extras such as extra yogurt or pickled cabbage, chilli sauce and hummus.

Spicy chicken couscous

Ingredients

250g couscous

3 tbsp olive oil

1 chopped onion

2 large sliced skinless boneless chicken breast fillets

85g blanched almonds

1 tbsp hot curry paste

100g halved ready-to-eat apricots

120g pack fresh coriander

Directions

STAGE 1

Prepare couscous with reduced salt chicken stock, according to the packet instructions. Heat olive oil in a pan and cook the onion for 2-3 mins until softened.

STAGE 2

Toss in chicken breast fillets and stir fry for 5-6 mins until tender. Add the blanched almonds and, when golden, stir in the hot curry paste and cook for 1 min more.

STAGE 3

Add the couscous along with the apricots and the coriander. Toss until hot then serve with plain yogurt if you like.

Vegetarian ramen

Ingredients

80g pack instant noodles (look for an Asian brand with a flavour like sesame)

2 spring onions, finely chopped

½ head pak choi

1 egg

1 tsp sesame seeds

chilli sauce, to serve

Directions

STAGE 1

Cook the noodles with the sachet of flavouring provided (or use stock instead of the sachet, if you have it). Add the spring onions and pak choi for the final min.

STAGE 2

Meanwhile, simmer the egg for 6 mins from boiling, run it under cold water to stop it cooking, then peel it. Toast the sesame seeds in a frying pan.

STAGE 3

Tip the noodles and greens into a deep bowl, halve the boiled egg and place on top. Sprinkle with sesame seeds, then drizzle with the sauce or sesame oil provided with the noodles, and chilli sauce, if using.

Bacon & mushroom pasta

Ingredients

400g penne (or other tube shape) pasta

250g pack chestnut or button mushrooms, wiped clean

8 rashers streaky bacon

4 tbsp pesto (fresh from the chiller cabinet if possible)

200ml carton 50% fat crème fraîche

handful basil leaves

Directions

STAGE 1

Cook the pasta in boiling water in a large non-stick saucepan according to pack instructions. Meanwhile, slice the mushrooms and snip the bacon into bite-size pieces with scissors or a sharp knife.

STAGE 2

Reserve a few drops of the cooking water in a cup or bowl, then drain the pasta and set aside. Fry the bacon and mushrooms in the same pan until golden, about 5 mins. Keep the heat high so the mushrooms fry in the bacon fat, rather than sweat.

STAGE 3

Tip the pasta and reserved water back into the pan and stir over the heat for 1 min. Take the pan off the heat, spoon in the pesto and crème fraîche and most of the basil and stir to combine. Sprinkle with the remaining basil to serve.

Black bean & tortilla soup

Ingredients

2 tbsp olive oil

1 chopped onion

2 chopped peppers

3 crushed garlic cloves

2 tsp ground cumin

1 tsp garlic granules

1 tsp chilli powder

2 tbsp tomato purée

1l veg stock

400g can chopped tomatoes

2 tbsp cornmeal or polenta

2 tbsp chopped pickled jalapeños

2 x 400g cans black beans

jalapeño brine

4 small corn tortillas

chopped coriander, avocado, crumbled feta and pumpkin seeds, to serve, if you like

Directions

STAGE 1

Heat the olive oil in a deep pan over a medium heat. Add the onion, peppers (any colour you like) and garlic cloves with a big pinch of salt. Cook for 10 mins, until starting to soften, then add the ground cumin, garlic granules and chilli powder along with the tomato purée. Cook for 5 mins, until the purée has caramelised.

STAGE 2

Pour in the veg stock, chopped tomatoes, cornmeal or polenta, chopped pickled jalapeños and black beans, along with the liquid. Add a splash of jalapeño brine and bring to a simmer. Cook for 45 mins, until thickened and reduced. Season, then scatter in the corn tortillas, cut into small strips. (Use flour tortillas if that's what you have.) Rest for 5 mins before serving. Serve with chopped coriander, avocado, crumbled feta and pumpkin seeds, if you like.

Orzo & chickpea soup

Ingredients

2 tbsp olive oil

1 onion, chopped

2 carrots, chopped

2 celery sticks, chopped

2 tbsp tomato purée

3 garlic cloves, chopped

3 rosemary or thyme sprigs

1 litre vegetable stock

400g can chopped tomatoes

400g can chickpeas

parmesan rind or vegetarian alternative (optional)

150g orzo

extra virgin olive oil, to serve

Directions

STAGE 1

Heat the olive oil in a deep pan over a medium-high heat and cook the onion, carrots and celery, including any leaves for 15 mins until softened. Stir in the tomato purée, garlic cloves and rosemary or thyme sprigs. Cook for a few minutes until the purée is caramelised. Pour in the stock, chopped tomatoes, chickpeas (and the liquid from the can) and parmesan rind, if you have one. Simmer 15 mins.

STAGE 2

Pour boiling water over the orzo in a heatproof bowl and set aside for 15 mins. Drain the orzo, add to the pan and cook for 5-8 mins until the orzo is tender. Fish out and discard the rosemary stalks and cheese rind, then season well. Drizzle over extra virgin olive oil and grated cheese to serve.

Spanish rice & prawn one-pot

Ingredients

1 onion, sliced

1 red and 1 green pepper, deseeded and sliced

50g chorizo, sliced

2 garlic cloves, crushed

1 tbsp olive oil

250g easy cook basmati rice (we used Tilda)

400g can chopped tomato

200g raw, peeled prawns, defrosted if frozen

Directions

STAGE 1

Boil the kettle. In a non-stick frying or shallow pan
with a lid, fry the onion, peppers, chorizo and garlic
in the oil over a high heat for 3 mins. Stir in the rice
and chopped tomatoes with 500ml boiling water,
cover, then cook over a high heat for 12 mins.

STAGE 2

Uncover, then stir – the rice should be almost tender.
Stir in the prawns, with a splash more water if the
rice is looking dry, then cook for another min until
the prawns are just pink and rice tender.

Ratatouille

Ingredients

2 large aubergines

4 small courgettes

2 red or yellow peppers

4 large ripe tomatoes

5 tbsp olive oil

supermarket pack or small bunch basil

1 medium onion, peeled and thinly sliced

3 garlic cloves, peeled and crushed

1 tbsp red wine vinegar

1 tsp sugar (any kind)

Directions

STAGE 1

Cut 2 large aubergines in half lengthways. Place them on the board, cut side down, slice in half lengthways again and then across into 1.5cm chunks. Cut the ends off 4 small courgettes, then across into 1.5cm slices.

STAGE 2

Peel 2 red or yellow peppers from stalk to bottom. Hold upright, cut around the stalk, then cut into 3 pieces. Cut away any membrane, then chop into bite-size chunks.

STAGE 3

Score a small cross on the base of each of 4 large ripe tomatoes, then put them into a heatproof bowl. Pour boiling water over, leave for 20 secs, then remove. Pour the water away, replace the tomatoes and cover with cold water. Leave to cool, then peel the skin away.

STAGE 4

Quarter the tomatoes, scrape away the seeds with a spoon, then roughly chop the flesh.

STAGE 5

Set a sauté pan over medium heat and when hot, pour in 2 tbsp olive oil. Brown the aubergines for 5 mins on each side until the pieces are soft. Set them aside.

STAGE 6

Fry the courgettes in another tbsp oil for 5 mins, until golden on both sides. Repeat with the peppers. Don't overcook the vegetables at this stage.

STAGE 7

Tear up the leaves from the bunch of basil and set aside. Cook 1 thinly sliced medium onion in the pan for 5 minutes. Add 3 crushed garlic cloves and fry for a further minute. Stir in 1 tbsp red wine vinegar and 1 tsp sugar, then tip in the tomatoes and half the basil.

STAGE 8

Return the vegetables to the pan with some salt and pepper and cook for 5 mins. Serve with basil.

Vegan leek & potato soup

Ingredients

1 tbsp rapeseed oil, plus a drizzle to serve (optional)

2 large garlic cloves, chopped

500g leeks, thinly sliced

500g potatoes, cut into cubes

500ml vegan vegetable stock, made with 1½ tsp bouillon powder

500ml unsweetened almond milk

chopped chives and bread, to serve

Directions

STAGE 1

Heat the oil in a large pan over a medium heat and fry the garlic and leeks, stirring, until the veg has started to soften. Add the potatoes and stock, then cover and simmer for 15 mins until the leeks and potatoes are soft.

STAGE 2

Pour in the almond milk, then remove from the heat and blitz using a hand blender until almost smooth, with a slightly chunky texture. Or, if you prefer, blitz until completely smooth. Reheat over a low heat if needed, then ladle into bowls and scatter with chives, drizzle with a little oil and serve with bread, if you like. Can be frozen for up to three months.

DINNER RECIPES FOR SPINAL STENOSIS

Air fryer buffalo cauliflower wings

Ingredients

1 tbsp sweet smoked paprika

1 tbsp ground cumin

½ tbsp garlic granules

50g plain flour

200g buttermilk (195ml)

1 medium cauliflower (around 750g), leaves removed and cut into florets

100g hot sauce

1 tbsp olive oil

1 tbsp honey or maple syrup

Directions

STAGE 1

Combine the paprika, cumin, garlic granules, flour, buttermilk and a good pinch of salt and freshly ground black pepper in a bowl and mix well to make a smooth batter. Add the cauliflower florets and mix to coat the cauliflower.

STAGE 2

Put the cauliflower florets in the air fryer basket in a single layer, shaking off any excess batter as you do so. You may need to cook in batches depending on the size of the basket. Cook on 200C for 18-20 mins, turning half way through, until browned on the edges.

STAGE 3

Meanwhile, combine the hot sauce, olive oil and honey or maple syrup, if using, in a large bowl. Add the cooked cauliflower and set aside while you cook your next batch, if necessary. Gently mix all of the cooked cauliflower and hot sauce to coat. Finally, return all of the cauliflower to your air fryer basket and cook for 6-9 mins until hot and well cooked through.

Spanish rice & prawn one-pot

Ingredients

1 onion, sliced

1 red and 1 green pepper, deseeded and sliced

50g chorizo, sliced

2 garlic cloves, crushed

1 tbsp olive oil

250g easy cook basmati rice (we used Tilda)

400g can chopped tomato

200g raw, peeled prawns, defrosted if frozen

Directions

STAGE 1

Boil the kettle. In a non-stick frying or shallow pan with a lid, fry the onion, peppers, chorizo and garlic in the oil over a high heat for 3 mins. Stir in the rice and chopped tomatoes with 500ml boiling water, cover, then cook over a high heat for 12 mins.

STAGE 2

Uncover, then stir – the rice should be almost tender. Stir in the prawns, with a splash more water if the rice is looking dry, then cook for another min until the prawns are just pink and rice tender.

Portobello jackfruit burgers

Ingredients

900g potatoes, cut into slim chips

3 tbsp rapeseed oil, plus a drop

8 large flat portobello mushrooms (600g), stalks removed

smoked paprika, for sprinkling

For the burgers

410g can jackfruit in water, drained

2 tsp tamari

400g chickpeas, well drained

1 tbsp tomato purée

2 garlic cloves, chopped

2 tbsp wholemeal spelt flour

For the tomato relish

4 vine tomatoes, finely chopped

2 tsp tomato purée

1 tsp balsamic vinegar

2 tbsp finely chopped red onion

1-2 tbsp chopped basil or coriander

Directions

STAGE 1

Heat the oven to 200C/180C fan/gas 6. Toss the chips in 2½ tbsp of the oil and spread out on a large non-stick baking sheet lined with baking parchment. Rub the outside of the mushrooms with a drop of oil, then arrange them on another baking sheet, rounded-side up, and put the chips and mushrooms in the oven for 20 mins. Turn the mushrooms and chips over after 10 mins.

STAGE 2

Meanwhile, squeeze as much juice as you can out of the jackfruit. The best way is to wrap it in kitchen paper, then squeeze with your hands. Trim off the feathery bits of jackfruit that look a bit like shredded meat, weigh out 75g and stir in the tamari sauce. Tip the remaining jackfruit into a bowl. Add the chickpeas, tomato purée and garlic and blitz together until smooth using a hand blender or use a food processor. Stir in the remaining jackfruit and shape into four burgers about the size of the mushrooms. Coat in the flour.

STAGE 3

Check the chips and mushrooms and cook for 5-10 mins longer if needed. Meanwhile, heat the remaining oil and fry two of the burgers for a few minutes each side until brown and heated through. To make the relish, put the chopped tomatoes in a bowl with the tomato purée, vinegar, onion and basil or coriander.

STAGE 4

To serve, sandwich two of the burgers between the mushrooms. If the mushrooms are very juicy, blot with a little kitchen paper first. Serve with half the chips, sprinkled with the paprika, and serve half the relish on the side. The remaining mushrooms, burgers and chips will keep for two days in the fridge. To serve again, warm the remaining mushrooms and burgers in a low oven, and heat the chips, uncovered, until piping hot.

Courgette curry with lemon rice

Ingredients

For the curry

1 tbsp olive oil

2 tbsp ginger, very finely chopped

1½ tsp cumin seeds

1-2 red chillies, deseeded and finely chopped

6 garlic cloves, crushed

450g baby potatoes, thickly sliced

2 tsp ground coriander

1 tsp ground turmeric

4 large vine tomatoes, roughly chopped

1 tbsp tomato purée

200ml stock, made with 1 tsp vegetable bouillon powder

1 cinnamon stick

500g medium-sized courgettes, thickly sliced

15g chopped fresh coriander

For the lemon rice

1 tbsp olive oil

½-1 tsp brown mustard seeds (optional)

240g brown basmati rice

½-1 tsp turmeric

12 curry leaves (optional)

400g can chickpeas, drained

2 tbsp lemon juice

Directions

STAGE 1

Heat the oil in a large frying pan and fry the ginger for 3 mins. Stir in the cumin seeds, chillies and garlic and cook briefly, then add the potatoes, ground coriander and turmeric, and stir well. Tip in the tomatoes, tomato purée and stock, then add the cinnamon, cover, and leave to simmer for 5 mins.

STAGE 2

Stir in the courgettes, then cover and cook for 10-12 mins until the courgettes are tender rather than soft. Stir in the fresh coriander.

STAGE 3

Meanwhile, heat the oil in a pan and stir in the mustard seeds, if using, and cook until you hear them pop. Stir in the rice, turmeric and curry leaves, if using, then pour in 1 litre boiling water. Simmer, covered, for 15 mins, then add the chickpeas and lemon juice, cover once again, and cook for 10 mins more until the water has been absorbed and the rice is tender.

Cod & prawn pie with saffron potatoes

Ingredients

1 tbsp olive oil

1 yellow and red pepper, both deseeded and finely chopped

2 large garlic cloves, chopped

2 bay leaves

1 tbsp smoked paprika

150ml vegetable stock, made with 2 tsp bouillon powder

500g carton passata

240g pack frozen raw, peeled, large wild red shrimp, defrosted

2 x 280g packs skinless cod loin, cut into large chunks

9 pitted green olives, quartered (we used Amfissa olives, as they have a firmer texture)

3 tbsp chopped flat-leaf parsley (optional)

320g broccoli florets or green beans

For the saffron potatoes

3 generous pinches of saffron threads (about ⅓ x 0.5g sachet)

1 ½ tbsp olive oil

2 large garlic cloves, finely grated

725g large potatoes (about 4), peeled and thinly sliced

Directions

STAGE 1

Heat the oven to 200C/180C fan/ gas 6. Warm the olive oil in a large non-stick pan over a medium heat and fry the peppers, garlic and bay leaves for 10 mins, stirring often until the peppers have softened.

STAGE 2

Meanwhile, prepare the saffron potatoes. Put the saffron threads in a small heatproof bowl with 1 tbsp boiling water, the olive oil and garlic, and stir well until the liquid turns yellow. Set aside. Bring a large pan of water to the boil, and cook the sliced potatoes for 5 mins until tender but not collapsing. Drain well.

STAGE 3

When the peppers have softened, sprinkle over the paprika and stir briefly, then pour in the stock and passata and cook for 5 mins more. Remove from the heat and stir in the shrimp, cod, olives and parsley, if using. Tip the stew into a large, shallow pie dish (ours was 30 x 20cm, and about 6.5cm deep).

STAGE 4

Arrange the potato slices over the stew in an even layer – they don't have to be neat – then generously brush over the saffron mixture.

STAGE 5

Bake the pie for 30-35 mins until bubbling at the edges and the fish is cooked through. When it's almost finished cooking, boil or steam the broccoli or green beans to serve alongside the pie.

Vegan biryani

Ingredients

240g brown basmati rice

1½ tbsp rapeseed oil

1 large onion (220g), finely chopped

1 cinnamon stick

1 red chilli, deseeded and finely chopped (optional)

3 large garlic cloves, finely chopped

20g fresh ginger, peeled and finely chopped

1½ tsp cumin seeds

1 large red pepper, deseeded and roughly chopped

1 large aubergine (320g), cut into cubes

2 tbsp curry powder

400g can chopped tomatoes

2 tsp vegan bouillon powder

320g small cauliflower florets

30g coriander, stems and leaves separated and chopped

40g flame raisins

50g unsalted cashew nuts, toasted

Directions

STAGE 1

Rinse the rice until the water runs clear, then cook in a pan of fresh cold water following pack instructions for about 20 mins, or until almost tender.

STAGE 2

Meanwhile, heat the oil in a large, deep frying pan over a medium heat and stir in the onion, cinnamon stick, chilli, garlic and ginger so they're coated in the oil. Scatter over the cumin seeds, cover and cook for 5 mins.

STAGE 3

Stir well, then add the pepper and aubergine, and cook, stirring for 3-5 mins, until the veg is starting to soften. Stir in the curry powder, then the tomatoes and bouillon. Tip in the cauliflower florets, coriander stems and raisins, then cover and simmer for 10 mins over a medium-low heat.

STAGE 4

Drain the rice, then tip it into the veg mixture and gently toss to combine. Cover and cook over a low heat for 8 mins until the rice and cauliflower are tender. Try not to add extra liquid, as you don't want the end result to be wet. Remove from the heat and leave to stand for 5 mins, then gently toss through the cashews and coriander leaves. Will keep chilled for two days. Leave to cool completely first. Reheat portions in the microwave until piping hot before serving.

Healthy ragu

Ingredients

1 tbsp rapeseed oil

2 large onions (320g), halved or quartered, then sliced

3 large garlic cloves, finely grated

500g 5% fat steak mince

500g carton passata

3 carrots (320g), finely chopped

1 tbsp thyme leaves

1 tbsp vegetable bouillon powder

½ tsp ground white pepper

200g frozen peas

4 jacket potatoes, to serve

Directions

STAGE 1

Heat the oil in a large non-stick pan over a medium-low heat and fry the onions for 10 mins, stirring occasionally until golden. Stir in the garlic, then add the mince and cook, breaking it up with a wooden spoon as you do, for a few minutes more until browned.

STAGE 2

Add the passata, carrots, thyme, bouillon powder and pepper, then cover and cook over a low heat for 25-30 mins, stirring occasionally until the meat is cooked and veg is tender. Add a splash of water to loosen, if you like, then stir in the peas and cook for 5-7 mins more until tender. Serve hot over jacket potatoes. Once completely cool, the mince sauce will keep frozen for up to three months. Defrost in the fridge overnight and reheat until piping hot.

Fajita chicken one-pot

Ingredients

2 tsp olive oil

200g cooking chorizo, roughly chopped

6 boneless and skinless chicken thighs, roughly chopped

2 red onions, roughly chopped

2 Romano peppers, roughly chopped

1½ tbsp fajita seasoning

400g can pinto beans, drained and rinsed

350g new potatoes, halved, or quartered if large

300ml chicken stock, made with 1 stock cube

3 corn on the cobs, halved or quartered

100g soured cream, to serve

handful of parsley, chopped, to serve (optional)

Directions

STAGE 1

Heat the oil in a large, lidded, heavy-based saucepan over a medium heat and fry the chorizo for 4 mins to release the oils and brown it a little. Remove to a plate using a slotted spoon and set aside. Fry the chicken for 5-6 mins until browned but not cooked all the way through. You may need to do this in batches. Remove with the slotted spoon and set aside with the chorizo.

STAGE 2

Add the onions and peppers to the pan and cook, stirring often for 6-8 mins until softened and starting to lightly brown. Use a wooden spoon to scrape up any caramelised bits on the bottom and mix them in. Stir in the fajita seasoning and cook for 30 seconds before returning the chorizo and chicken to the pan.

STAGE 3

Season with salt and freshly ground black pepper and give everything a good stir. Tip in the pinto beans and potatoes, stir to coat well, then pour in the stock, topping up with water if it doesn't cover the chicken and veg. Bring to a simmer, reduce the heat a little and put the lid on. Simmer gently for 10 mins. Give everything a stir, then sit the corn on the cobs on top.

STAGE 4

Return the lid to the pan and cook for a further 15 mins. Serve in large bowls, each topped with a spoonful of soured cream and a scattering of chopped parsley, if you like.

Kale soup

Ingredients

2 tbsp rapeseed oil

3 onions (320g), finely chopped

3 garlic cloves, finely grated

125g celery, chopped

2 yellow peppers, deseeded and diced

2 tsp smoked paprika

400g can chopped tomatoes

2 tsp dried oregano

1 litre hot vegetable stock, made with 3 tsp bouillon
powder

150g wholemeal penne

200g green beans, trimmed and cut into short lengths

200g cavolo nero (kale), thinly sliced

160g cherry tomatoes

30g pack of basil, chopped

80g vegetarian Italian-style hard cheese, finely grated

Directions

STAGE 1

Heat the oil in a large pan over a medium heat and fry the onions and garlic for 5 mins, then add the celery and peppers. Fry for another 5 mins, adding the smoked paprika in the last minute. Stir in the tomatoes, oregano and stock. Bring to the boil.

STAGE 2

Tip in the penne, green beans and kale, bring back to the boil and cook over a medium heat for 10 mins. Stir in the cherry tomatoes and basil, and cook for a few minutes more until the tomatoes have burst.

STAGE 3

To serve, spoon two portions of the soup into shallow bowls and sprinkle over half the cheese. Keep the remainder for another day. Will keep chilled in an airtight container for up to four days or frozen for up to three months. Reheat in a pan over a low-medium heat until piping hot, then serve with the remaining cheese.

Spinach crespolini

Ingredients

50g spelt wholemeal flour

1 egg

100ml milk

½ tsp rapeseed oil

250g baby spinach

generous grating of nutmeg

1 large garlic clove, finely grated

80g ricotta

2 tbsp vegetarian Italian-style hard cheese, finely grated

For the sauce

400g can chopped tomatoes

10g basil

½ tsp vegetable bouillon powder

1 garlic clove, crushed

For the salad

2 tsp balsamic vinegar

1 small red onion (about 80g), finely chopped

80g diced celery

3 handfuls of rocket

160g cherry tomatoes

Directions

STAGE 1

Whisk the flour and egg together, then gradually whisk in the milk to create a smooth pancake-style batter. Pour into a jug.

STAGE 2

Heat the oil in a 19cm non-stick pan over a medium heat, tip in a quarter of the batter, and swirl to cover the base. Cook briefly until just set, then flip over using a palette knife and cook the other side until just golden. Lift onto a plate, then repeat with the remaining batter to make four pancakes in total.

STAGE 3

Meanwhile, heat a second large non-stick pan over a medium heat and cook the spinach, nutmeg and garlic for about 5 mins, stirring with a wooden spoon until the spinach has completely wilted. Remove from the heat and cool slightly, then beat in the ricotta. Spoon a quarter of the spinach filling down the centre of each pancake, then roll up into a sausage and arrange snugly in an ovenproof dish. Heat the oven to 200C/180C fan/gas 6.

STAGE 4

To make the sauce, put the canned tomatoes, basil, bouillon and garlic in a bowl, and blitz using a hand blender until completely smooth (or do this in a jug blender). Pour the sauce over the pancakes and scatter over the cheese. Bake for 30 mins until browned and bubbling at the edges. For the salad, combine the vinegar, onion and celery. Just before serving, toss the onion mixture with the rocket and tomatoes, and serve with the filled pancakes.

Miso salmon with ginger noodles

Ingredients

2 nests wholemeal noodles (100g)

1 ½ tsp brown miso

2 tsp balsamic vinegar

½ tsp smoked paprika

2 skinless wild salmon fillets (230g)

1 tbsp rapeseed oil

30g ginger, cut into matchsticks

1 green pepper, deseeded and cut into strips

2 leeks (165g), thinly sliced

3 garlic cloves, finely grated

160g baby spinach

Directions

STAGE 1

Put the noodles in a bowl, cover with boiling water and set aside to soften. Heat the grill to medium and place a piece of foil on the grill rack. Mix 1 tsp of the miso with the vinegar, paprika and 1 tbsp water. Spread over the salmon and grill for 6-8 mins until flaky and cooked.

STAGE 2

Heat the oil in a wok and stir-fry the ginger, pepper and leeks over a high heat for a few mins until softened. Add the garlic and cook for 1 min more. Drain the noodles, reserve 2 tbsp water and mix with the remaining miso.

STAGE 3

Add the drained noodles, miso liquid and spinach to the wok and toss over the heat until the spinach wilts. Pile onto plates, top with the salmon and any juices and serve.

Vegetarian enchiladas

Ingredients

1 tsp olive oil

2 onions, chopped

280g carrots, grated

2-3 tsp chilli powder (mild or hot, according to your taste)

2 x 400g cans chopped tomatoes

2 x 400g cans pulses in water, drained (we used mixed beans and lentils)

6 small wholemeal tortillas

200g low-fat natural yogurt

50g extra-mature cheddar cheese (or veg alternative), finely grated

Directions

STAGE 1

Heat the oil in a large frying pan. Cook the onions and carrots for 5-8 mins until soft – add a splash of water if they start to stick. Sprinkle in the chilli powder and cook for 1 min more. Pour in the tomatoes and pulses and bring to the boil. Turn down the heat and simmer for 5-10 mins, stirring occasionally, until thickened. Remove from the heat and season well.

STAGE 2

Heat grill to high. Spread a spoonful of the bean chilli over a large ovenproof dish. Lay each tortilla onto a board, fill with a few tbsp of chilli mixture, fold over the ends and roll up to seal. Place them into the ovenproof dish. Spoon the remaining chilli on top.

STAGE 3

Mix the yogurt and grated cheese together with some seasoning, and spoon over the enchiladas. Grill for a few mins until the top is golden and bubbling. Serve with a green salad.

Prawn jambalaya

Ingredients

1 tbsp rapeseed oil

1 onion, chopped

3 celery sticks, sliced

100g wholegrain basmati rice

1 tsp mild chilli powder

1 tbsp ground coriander

½ tsp fennel seeds

400g can chopped tomatoes

1 tsp vegetable bouillon powder

1 yellow pepper, roughly chopped

2 garlic cloves, chopped

1 tbsp fresh thyme leaves

150g pack small prawns, thawed if frozen

3 tbsp chopped parsley

Directions

STAGE 1

Heat the oil in a large, deep frying pan. Add the onion and celery, and fry for 5 mins to soften. Add the rice and spices, and pour in the tomatoes with just under 1 can of water. Stir in the bouillon powder, pepper, garlic and thyme.

STAGE 2

Cover the pan with a lid and simmer for 30 mins until the rice is tender and almost all the liquid has been absorbed. Stir in the prawns and parsley, cook briefly to heat through, then serve.

Creamy chicken stew

Ingredients

3 leeks, halved and finely sliced

2 tbsp olive oil, plus extra if needed

1 tbsp butter

8 small chicken thighs

500ml chicken stock

1 tbsp Dijon mustard

75g crème fraîche

200g frozen peas

3 tbsp dried or fresh breadcrumbs

small bunch of parsley, finely chopped

Directions

STAGE 1

Tip the leeks and oil into a flameproof casserole dish on a low heat, add the butter and cook everything very gently for 10 mins or until the leeks are soft.

STAGE 2

Put the chicken, skin-side down, in a large non-stick frying pan on a medium heat, cook until the skin browns, then turn and brown the other side. You shouldn't need any oil but if the skin starts to stick, add a little. Add the chicken to the leeks, leaving behind any fat in the pan.

STAGE 3

Add the stock to the dish and bring to a simmer, season well, cover and cook for 30 mins on low. Stir in the mustard, crème fraîche and peas and bring to a simmer. You should have quite a bit of sauce.

STAGE 4

When you're ready to serve, put the grill on. Mix the breadcrumbs and parsley, sprinkle them over the chicken and grill until browned.

Chicken & sweetcorn soup

Ingredients

1 chicken carcass

4 thin slices fresh ginger, plus 1 tbsp finely grated

2 onions, quartered

3 garlic cloves, finely grated

2 tsp apple cider vinegar

325g can sweetcorn

3 spring onions, whites thinly sliced, greens sliced at
an angle

100g cooked chicken, shredded

2 tsp tamari

2 eggs, beaten

few drops sesame oil, to serve (optional)

Directions

STAGE 1

Boil a large kettle of water. Break the carcass into a big non-stick pan and add the ginger slices, onion and two-thirds of the garlic. Cook, stirring, for about 2 mins – the meat will stick to the base of the pan, but this will add to the flavour. Pour in 1.5 litres of boiling water, stir in the vinegar, then cover and simmer for 2 hrs.

STAGE 2

Put a large sieve over a bowl and pour through the contents of the pan. Measure the liquid in the bowl – you want around 450ml. If you have too much, return to the pan and boil with the lid off to reduce it. Transfer the onion from the sieve to a bowl with three-quarters of the sweetcorn. Blitz until smooth with a hand blender.

STAGE 3

Return the broth to the pan, and tip in the puréed corn, remaining sweetcorn and garlic, the grated ginger, the whites of the spring onions and the chicken. Simmer for 5 mins, then stir in the tamari. Turn off the heat, and quickly drizzle in the egg, stirring a little to create egg threads. Season with pepper, then ladle into the bowls. Top with the spring onion greens and a few drops of sesame oil, if using.

SNACK RECIPES FOR SPINAL STENOSIS

Mini pumpkin & feta pies

Ingredients

450g butternut squash or pumpkin peeled and cut into 2cm chunks (prepared weight)

2 garlic cloves

2 tbsp olive oil

1 small onion, finely chopped

250g plain flour, plus extra for dusting

½ tsp ground turmeric

125g cold butter, cut into small pieces, plus extra for the tin

2 egg yolks plus 1 whole egg, beaten

grating of nutmeg

½ tsp chilli flakes (optional)

200g feta, crumbled

Directions

STAGE 1

Heat the oven to 200C/180C fan/gas 6. Tip the squash and unpeeled garlic into a roasting tin, drizzle with 1 tbsp oil, season and toss to coat. Roast for 30 mins, stirring halfway through, until soft. Remove from the oven and leave to cool.

STAGE 2

Meanwhile, cook the onion in a frying pan over a medium heat with the remaining 1 tbsp oil for 8-10 mins until tender and slightly golden. Leave to cool.

STAGE 3

Tip the flour, turmeric and a pinch of salt into a food processor. Add the butter and whizz until the mixture resembles fine crumbs. Add the egg yolks and 2 tsp cold water, and blitz again until the mixture starts to clump together. Squeeze it between your fingers – if it sticks together, tip the mixture onto a work surface. If it's too dry, add more water, 1 tsp at a time. Knead the pastry a few times just to bring it together, but don't overwork it. Shape into two circles, one slightly smaller than the other, then wrap in baking parchment and chill in the fridge for at least 20 mins.

STAGE 4

Squeeze the garlic from its skins into the roasted squash and mash together. Add the fried onion, grate over some nutmeg, tip in the chilli flakes, if using, and feta, and mix.

STAGE 5

Butter six holes of a muffin tin and line each with a strip of baking parchment that overhangs the top. Roll the larger circle of pastry out on a lightly floured surface to the thickness of a £1 coin. Use a 10cm cutter to stamp out six circles (you may need to re-roll the pastry to get all six). Press the pastry circles into the prepared muffin tin, patching any cracks with the pastry offcuts. Spoon in the squash filling.

STAGE 6

Roll the remaining pastry circle out as you did the large one, but use an 8cm cutter to cut out six lids. Cut spooky pumpkin faces into the lids using a small, sharp knife. Press the lids over the pies in the tin and brush with the beaten egg. Bake for 40 mins until golden brown, then leave to cool for 10 mins in the tin before lifting out. Eat hot or leave to cool completely. Will keep in an airtight container in the fridge for up to two days or the freezer for up to two months. Reheat in a low oven for 10 mins, if you like.

Homemade toffee apples

Ingredients

8 Granny Smith apples

400g golden caster sugar

1 tsp vinegar

4 tbsp golden syrup

Directions

STAGE 1

Place the apples in a large bowl, then cover with boiling water (you may have to do this in 2 batches). This will remove the waxy coating and help the caramel to stick. Dry thoroughly and twist off any stalks. Push a wooden skewer or lolly stick into the stalk end of each apple.

STAGE 2

Lay out a sheet of baking parchment and place the apples on this, close to your stovetop. Tip the sugar into a pan along with 100ml water and set over a medium heat. Cook for 5 mins until the sugar dissolves, then stir in the vinegar and syrup. Set a sugar thermometer in the pan and boil to 150C or 'hard crack' stage. If you don't have a thermometer you can test the toffee by pouring a little into a bowl of cold water. It should harden instantly and, when removed, be brittle and easy to break. If you can still squish the toffee, continue to boil it.

STAGE 3

Working quickly and carefully, dip and twist each apple in the hot toffee until covered, let any excess drip away, then place on the baking parchment to harden. You may have to heat the toffee a little if the temperature drops and it starts to feel thick and viscous. Leave the toffee to cool before eating. Can be made up to 2 days in advance, stored in a dry place.

Next level scotch eggs

Ingredients

6 eggs, at room temperature

5 Cumberland sausages (about 350g)

2 rashers smoked streaky bacon, finely chopped or minced

1 litre sunflower oil, for frying

For the coating

2 eggs, beaten

100g plain flour

2 tsp English mustard powder

50g packet of salt and vinegar crisps, crushed

100g panko breadcrumbs

Directions

STAGE 1

Bring a pan of salted water to the boil, carefully drop in the eggs and set a timer for 7 mins. After 7 mins, immediately scoop out the eggs using a slotted spoon and transfer to a bowl of iced water, cracking the shells a little with the spoon as you do (this makes them easier to peel later). Leave to cool completely, then peel and set aside.

STAGE 2

Squeeze the sausagemeat from the skins into a small bowl, add the bacon and mix to combine. For the coating, tip the beaten egg into a shallow container. Combine the flour and mustard powder in a second, and stir together the crushed crisps and panko breadcrumbs in a third.

STAGE 3

Divide the sausage mixture into six rough portions. Lay a sheet of baking parchment on the work surface, then drop a portion of the meat into the middle of the parchment. Top with a second sheet of baking parchment and flatten the meat into a disc using your palm. Remove the top sheet of parchment. Roll one of the eggs in the flour mix, then place in the middle of the sausagemeat disc. Use the parchment to help you wrap the meat around the egg so it's completely encased, trimming any excess from the top and bottom. Repeat with the rest of the eggs and meat. Dip the sausage-coated eggs back in the flour mix, then the egg, then the crumbs, back into the egg, then finally, in the crumbs again. Can be prepared up to a few hours ahead and chilled until ready to fry.

STAGE 4

Heat a 5cm depth of oil in a wok, wide saucepan or deep-fat fryer until it reaches 160C or until a cube of bread dropped in turns golden in 10 seconds. Lower in as many eggs as you can, being careful not to overcrowd the pan, and fry for 6-8 mins, gently turning until golden and crisp on all sides. Drain on kitchen paper, leave to cool a little, then serve.

Double ginger cookies

Ingredients

350g plain flour

1 tbsp ground ginger

1 tsp bicarbonate of soda

175g light muscovado sugar

100g butter, chopped

8 pieces of stem ginger, chopped (not too finely), plus thin slices, to decorate (optional)

1 large egg

4 tbsp golden syrup

200g bar dark chocolate, chopped

Directions

STAGE 1

Mix the flour, ground ginger, bicarbonate of soda, 1/2 tsp salt and sugar in a bowl, then rub in the butter to make crumbs. Stir in the chopped stem ginger.

STAGE 2

Beat together the egg and syrup, pour into the dry Ingredients and stir, then knead with your hands to make a dough. Cut the dough in half and shape each piece into a thick sausage about 6cm across, making sure that the ends are straight. Wrap in cling film and chill for 20 mins. You can now freeze all or part of the dough for 2 months.

STAGE 3

Heat oven to 180C/160C fan/gas 4 and line 2 baking sheets with baking parchment. Thickly slice each sausage into 12 and put the slices on the baking sheets, spacing them well apart and reshaping any, if necessary, to make rounds. Bake for 12 mins, then leave to cool for a few mins to harden before transferring to a wire rack to cool completely.

STAGE 4

Melt the chocolate in a bowl over a pan of gently simmering water, making sure that the water isn't touching the bottom of the bowl. Dip half of each cookie into the chocolate – you may need to spoon it over when you get to the final few. Decorate with a slice of ginger, if you like, and leave to set. Will keep for 1 week in an airtight container.

Flat apple & vanilla tart

Ingredients

375g pack puff pastry, preferably all-butter

5 large eating apples - Cox's, russets or Elstar

juice of 1 lemon

25g butter, cut into small pieces

3 tsp vanilla sugar or 1 tsp vanilla extract

1 tbsp caster sugar

3 rounded tbsp apricot conserve

Directions

STAGE 1

Heat oven to 220C/fan 200C/gas 7. Roll out the pastry and trim to a round about 35cm across. Transfer to a baking sheet lined with parchment paper.

STAGE 2

Peel, core and thinly slice the apples and toss in the lemon juice. Spread over the pastry to within 2cm of the edges. Curl up the edges slightly to stop the juices running off.

STAGE 3

Dot the top with the butter and sprinkle with vanilla and caster sugar. Bake for 15-20 mins until the apples are tender and the pastry crisp.

STAGE 4

Warm the conserve and brush over the apples and pastry edge. Serve hot with vanilla ice cream or crème fraîche.

Homemade vegan bagels

Ingredients

7g sachet dried yeast

4 tbsp sugar

2 tsp salt

450g bread flour

poppy, fennel and/or sesame seeds to sprinkle on top
(optional)

Directions

STAGE 1

Tip the yeast and 1 tbsp sugar into a large bowl, and
pour over 100ml warm water. Leave for 10 mins until
the mixture becomes frothy.

STAGE 2

Pour 200ml warm water into the bowl, then stir in the
salt and half the flour. Keep adding the remaining

flour (you may not have to use it all) and mixing with your hands until you have a soft but not sticky dough. Then knead for 10 mins until the dough feels smooth and elastic. Shape into a ball and put in a clean, lightly oiled bowl. Cover loosely and leave in a warm place until doubled in size, about 1hr.

STAGE 3

Heat the oven to 220C/200C fan/gas 7. On a lightly floured surface, divide the dough into 10 pieces, each about 85g. Shape each piece into a flattish ball, then take a wooden spoon and use the handle to make a hole in the middle of each ball. Slip the spoon into the hole, then twirl the bagel around the spoon to make a hole about 3cm wide. Cover the bagel loosely while you shape the remaining dough.

STAGE 4

Meanwhile, bring a large pan of water to the boil and tip in the remaining sugar. Slip the bagels into the boiling water – no more than four at a time. Cook for

1-2 mins, turning over in the water until the bagels have puffed slightly and a skin has formed. Remove with a slotted spoon and drain away any excess water. Sprinkle over your choice of topping and place on a baking tray lined with parchment. Bake in the oven for 25 mins until browned and crisp – the bases should sound hollow when tapped. Leave to cool on a wire rack, then serve with your favourite filling.

Carrot & pecan muffins

Ingredients

2 x 400g can cannellini beans in water, drained

2 tsp ground cinnamon

100g porridge oats

4 large eggs

2 tbsp rapeseed oil

4 tbsp maple syrup

2 tsp vanilla extract

zest 1 large orange

170g carrot, coarsely grated

100g raisins

80g pecan halves, 12 reserved, the rest roughly chopped

2 tsp baking powder

Directions

STAGE 1

Heat oven to 180C/160C fan/gas 4 and line a 12-hole muffin tin with paper cases. Tip the beans into a bowl and add the cinnamon, oats, eggs, oil, maple syrup, vanilla extract and orange zest. Blitz with a hand blender until really smooth – the beans and oats should be ground down as much as possible.

STAGE 2

Stir in the carrot, raisins, chopped pecans and baking powder, and mix well. Spoon into the muffin cases – use a large ice cream scoop if you have one, to get nice even muffins.

STAGE 3

Top each muffin with a reserved pecan and bake for 20 mins until set and light brown. Cool on a wire rack. Will keep in the fridge for a few days, or freeze for 6 weeks; thaw at room temperature.

Smoked mackerel risotto

Ingredients

1 tbsp butter

1 onion, finely chopped

250g risotto rice

100ml white wine

1l vegetable stock

1 x 240 pack smoked mackerel

2 spring onions, sliced

100g bag fresh spinach

Directions

STAGE 1

Heat the butter in a large frying pan. Tip in the onion, then fry gently for 5 mins until softened. Stir in the rice and mix until coated in the butter, then pour in the wine and let it bubble until it's almost all disappeared.

STAGE 2

Pour in half the stock, give it a good stir, then leave to gently cook for 10 mins. Add half of the remaining stock, stir again and cook for 5 mins more. Keep adding stock and cooking until the rice is tender.

STAGE 3

Peel the skin off the mackerel, scrape away any dark brown flesh, then flake. Stir into the rice with the spring onions and spinach, then cook just until the spinach has wilted slightly. Serve straight away.

Puff pastry pizzas

Ingredients

320g sheet ready-rolled light puff pastry

6 tbsp tomato purée

1 tbsp tomato ketchup

1 tsp dried oregano

75g mozzarella or cheddar

For the topping

sweetcorn, olives, peppers, red onion, cherry tomatoes, spinach, basil

Directions

STAGE 1

Heat the oven to 200C/180C fan/gas 6, or if using an air-fryer, heat it to 180C for 4 mins. Unroll the pastry, cut into six squares and arrange over two baking trays lined with baking parchment. Use a cutlery knife to score a 1cm border around the edge of each pastry square. Bake in the oven for 15 mins, until puffed up but not cooked through. Or, if using an air-fryer, bake the batch for 8 mins. You might need to do this in two batches.

STAGE 2

While the pastry cooks, make the sauce and prepare your toppings. Mix the tomato purée, tomato ketchup, oregano and 1 tbsp water. Grate the cheese and chop any veg or herbs you want to put on top into small pieces. Set aside.

STAGE 3

Remove the pastry from the oven or air-fryer and squash down the middles with the back of a spoon. Divide the sauce between the pastry squares and spread it out to the puffed-up edges. Sprinkle with the cheese, then add your toppings. Bake for another 5-8 mins in the oven or 5 mins in the air-fryer and serve.

Sweetcorn fritters

Ingredients

150g self-raising flour

1 tsp baking powder

1 tsp smoked paprika

160ml whole milk

1 egg

550g sweetcorn

2 spring onions, chopped, plus a little extra cut into thin strips to serve (optional)

10g sliced chives

handful of parsley, chopped

rapeseed oil, for frying

Directions

STAGE 1

Mix the flour, baking powder, paprika and milk together in a large bowl. Mix in the egg, followed by the sweetcorn, chopped spring onions, chives, parsley, 1 tsp salt and some freshly ground black pepper.

STAGE 2

Heat a 1cm depth of oil in a frying pan over a medium heat until a small amount of the fritter mixture sizzles when dropped in. For larger fritters, drop 2 heaped tablespoons of the mixture into the pan at a time in a clockwise direction (this will help you remember the order they were added to the pan, so you can flip them at the right stage). For smaller fritters, do the same, but with 1 heaped tablespoon of mixture at a time.

STAGE 3

After 2 mins, flip the fritters over in the same order they were added to the pan. Cook for another 2 mins, continuing to turn every now and then to ensure both sides are evenly golden brown. When ready, the fritters should be darker brown with crispy pieces of corn at the edges – be careful, as some of the kernels may burst during the cooking process. Remove to a wire rack and pat away any excess oil using kitchen paper. Serve straightaway with a few strips of spring onion scattered over, if you like.

Cheese-stuffed garlic dough balls with a tomato sauce dip

Ingredients

50g butter, cubed

300g strong white bread flour

7g sachet fast-action dried yeast

1 tbsp caster sugar

200g block mozzarella, cut into 1.5cm cubes

65g gruyère, coarsely grated (optional)

For the garlic butter

100g butter

2 garlic cloves, crushed

1 rosemary sprig, leaves picked and finely chopped

For the tomato sauce dip

1 tbsp olive oil, plus extra for the bowl and baking
sheet

1 garlic clove, sliced

250g passata

1 tsp red wine vinegar

1 tsp caster sugar

pinch of chilli flakes

½ small bunch of basil, torn, plus extra to serve

Directions

STAGE 1

Heat 175ml water in a saucepan until steaming, then add the butter. Remove from the heat and leave to cool until the mixture is just warm (it should not be hot). Combine the flour, yeast, sugar and 1 tsp salt in a large bowl or stand mixer. Add the cooled butter mixture, and mix to a soft dough using a wooden spoon or the mixer. Knead for 10 mins by hand (or 5 mins using a mixer) until the dough feels bouncy and smooth. Transfer to an oiled bowl and cover with a clean tea towel. Leave somewhere warm to rise for 1½-2 hrs, or until doubled in size. Alternatively, leave to prove in the fridge overnight.

STAGE 2

Oil and line a baking sheet with baking parchment. Knock the air out of the dough, then knead again for several minutes. Flatten a small piece of dough (about 20g) into a disc, and put a cube of the mozzarella and a pinch of the gruyère into the middle of the disc. Enclose the cheeses with the dough, then roll into a ball. Transfer to the prepared baking sheet. Repeat with the remaining cheese and dough, placing the dough balls ½cm apart on the baking sheet – they should be just touching after proving. Cover with a clean tea towel and leave somewhere warm to rise for 30 mins.

STAGE 3

Meanwhile, make the garlic butter. Melt the butter in a small pan over a low heat, then stir in the garlic and rosemary. Remove from the heat and set aside until needed. Heat the oven to 180C/160C fan/gas 4. Brush the risen dough balls with the garlic butter, then bake for 25-30 mins until the dough balls are cooked through and the middles are oozing.

STAGE 4

While the dough balls are baking, make the tomato sauce dip. Heat the oil in a saucepan and fry the garlic for 30 seconds. Tip in the passata, vinegar, sugar and chilli flakes, and simmer for 10 mins until thickened. Season to taste and stir in the basil. Brush the warm dough balls with any remaining garlic butter, then serve with the tomato sauce dip on the side for dunking.

Instant berry banana slush

Ingredients

2 ripe bananas

200g frozen berry mix (blackberries, raspberries and currants)

Directions

STAGE 1

Slice the bananas into a bowl and add the frozen berry mix. Blitz with a stick blender to make a slushy ice and serve straight away in two glasses with spoons.

Ricotta and basil pizza

Ingredients

1 onion, finely chopped

2 yellow peppers, roughly chopped

1 tsp olive oil

2 x 400g/14oz cans chopped tomatoes

500g bag mixed grain or granary bread mix

plain flour, for dusting

10 cherry tomatoes, halved or whole

250g tub ricotta

a few basil leaves, to serve

Directions

STAGE 1

Heat oven to 220C/fan 200C/gas 6. Soften the onion and peppers in the oil in a large pan for a few mins. Pour in the tomatoes, season, then simmer for 10 mins.

STAGE 2

Meanwhile, make up the bread mix according to pack instructions, then bring the dough together and knead a couple of times. Flour a large baking sheet and roll out the dough into a rectangle roughly 25 x 35cm. Bake for 5 mins on a shelf at the top of the oven until firm.

STAGE 3

Remove from the oven, spread with the sauce, add the cherry tomatoes, then dollop over spoonfuls of the ricotta. Bake for 10 mins more until the base is golden and crisp. Scatter with basil and serve straight away with a green salad.

Caramelised mushroom tartlets

Ingredients

2 tbsp olive oil

1 onion, chopped

1 tbsp golden caster sugar

250g chestnut mushrooms, cleaned and thinly sliced

1 garlic clove, crushed

3-4 tbsp thyme leaves, finely chopped

butter, for spreading

12 slices of thin sliced white sandwich bread

100g grated gruyère or cheddar, for sprinkling

Directions

STAGE 1

Heat the oil in a generous frying pan, add the onion and fry over moderate heat for about 7 mins until soft and golden. Stir in the sugar and seasoning, turn up the heat and add the mushrooms. Sizzle for 5 mins until you have driven off any moisture and the mushrooms are golden. Stir in the garlic for a few further mins, until fragrant, then turn off the heat and stir in most of the thyme (save some for sprinkling). The mushroom mix can be chilled at this point.

STAGE 2

To make the tartlet bases, cut 7-8cm circles out of the bread using a cookie cutter or glass. Butter one side and stick buttered-side down into a 12-hole tartlet tin. Freeze any leftovers to make breadcrumbs.

STAGE 3

When ready to bake, heat oven to 220C/200 fan/gas 7. Divide the mushroom mixture between the tartlets and top with a sprinkle of cheese. Don't be too tidy about this – any cheese on the tin will form a lacy edge to the tartlets. Bake for 10-15 mins until golden and bubbling. Sprinkle over the reserved herbs and serve.

PART V: Conclusion

In wrapping up, while diet isn't a magic fix for spinal stenosis, it's a critical piece of the puzzle for managing symptoms and improving daily life with this condition.

Embracing an anti-inflammatory diet packed with fruits, veggies, lean proteins, and good fats can really dial down inflammation and ease the pain linked to spinal stenosis. Plus, keeping a healthy weight through smart eating can take some pressure off the spine and slow down how fast the condition worsens.

Just remember, it's super important to team up with a healthcare expert or a dietitian to craft a diet plan that fits your unique needs and health situation. By blending a balanced diet with other treatments like physical therapy and meds prescribed by your doc, folks dealing with spinal stenosis can really boost their health and quality of life.

www.ingramcontent.com/pod-product-compliance
Lightning Source LLC
Chambersburg PA
CBHW061036250726
48653CB00001B/113